EKG Interpretation

Making EKG/ECG Interpretation Easy!

Table of Contents

Introduction

Thank you for taking the time to read this book about EKG/ECG interpretation! Whether you are studying to interpret Electrocardiograms, or if you simply want to better understand your own diagnosis and results, this book will be able to help.

In the following chapters, you will learn about what en EKG is, the different types you may encounter, and how they work. Most importantly, you will learn about the different conditions that an EKG can help to diagnose, and how to diagnose them.

Finally, you will learn about the implications of each diagnosis, and what steps may be taken post-diagnosis in order to improve or alleviate those conditions entirely.

This book doesn't aim to give you medical advice to act upon, but rather is exists to serve as a guide to Electrocardiograms for the layperson, or anyone who needs an additional study resource.

Once again, thanks for choosing this book, I hope you find it to be helpful!

Chapter 1: Definition of Electrocardiogram

What is an Electrocardiogram?

An electrocardiogram, also known as EKG or ECG, is a diagnostic tool used to record the muscular and electrical functions of the heart. This test monitors the status of the heart in many situations and detects heart problems.

With every beat of the heart, a "wave" or electrical impulse travels through the heart and causes the muscle to pump and squeeze blood from the heart. The EKG/ECG measures the rhythm and rate of the heartbeat, and also provides indirect proof of the heart muscle's blood flow.

How Is It Done?

EKG/ECG tests are often performed in a hospital room, a doctor's office, or a specialized clinic. Ambulances and operating rooms are also equipped with an EKG/ECG as standard equipment. An electrocardiogram is quite a simple test to perform, but the interpretation of the EKG/ECG tracing requires an enormous amount of training.

EKG/ECG tests are painless and noninvasive, and render quick results. To detect the electrical activities of the heart, sensors (electrodes or patches) with adhesive pads are attached to the chest, arms, and legs of the patient during an EKG/ECG test. Typically, these electrodes are attached for only a few minutes.

For a routine EKG/ECG, a standardized system has been created for the placement of the electrodes. It takes 10 electrodes to have a view of 12 areas of the heart. Six electrodes are placed on the chest, and one on each arm and leg. The signals from all the electrodes are recorded on the ECG machine, which also prints the tracings to a paper.

Newer ECG machines are now equipped with video screens that can help the doctor, nurse, or technician to determine whether the quality of the ECG tracings is sufficient, or if the test must be repeated. There are now ECG machines that have computer programs to help interpret the ECG results, but they may not be completely accurate.

In some cases, the physician may have to evaluate the heart from various angles after the first ECG. The chest leads will then be attached on the back, or across the right chest wall.

In comparison to EKG/ECG, a heart monitor only uses three electrodes – one each on the left chest, left arm, and right arm. It only measures the rhythm and rate of the heartbeat. This type of monitoring is not a complete electrocardiogram.

How to Prepare for an EKG

Although there are no actual preparations necessary before having an EKG, you can still do some things to prepare yourself for it, including:

- Wear a shirt that can be easily removed to place the electrodes on your chest.

- The skin must be dry and clean to avoid electrical interference to obtain an acceptable ECG tracing or interpretation. You may have to aggressively towel off your skin.

- If you are a male, you may have to shave your chest hair to allow better connection of the electrodes on your skin.

- Avoid ankle-length legwear because there are electrodes that will be placed on your legs.

- Avoid lotions and oily skin cream on the day of the EKG because they can make the electrodes resist contact with your skin.

- Before taking the EKG, inform your doctor about any supplements or medications you are taking as they may have an effect on the results of the test.

Will You Need More Tests After the Initial EKG?

You may need to do other tests later on, depending on the EKG findings and the symptoms you feel. For instance, if the test result is normal after taking an ECG at rest, but you feel chest pain or shortness of breath when walking uphill or upstairs, you will most likely be recommended to take a stress test or exercise EKG. This test will be recorded while you are walking on a treadmill.

Consequently, this test may give rise to further evaluations, such as a coronary angiogram or CT angiogram to check if there is anything that obstructs blood flow to your heart.

If you are experiencing palpitations or a rapid, irregular heartbeat, you may then be asked to take a longer EKG recording to find out if the palpitations are because of an abnormal heart rhythm. The recording may last for more than a few days, and you will have to use a small wearable EKG monitor.

Basic Anatomy of the Heart

There are four chambers of the heart: the right and left ventricle and the right and left atrium.

The two atria function as receiving chambers for blood that enters the heart, while the ventricles pump blood out of the heart.

This is how the blood flows throughout the body:

- Oxygen-rich blood that comes from the lungs goes into the left atrium via the pulmonary veins.

- The blood flows into the left ventricle and is then pumped into the aorta and circulated to the other parts of the body. This blood supplies cells and organs with nutrients and oxygen necessary for metabolism.

- The blood that goes back to the heart is poor in oxygen and brings along carbon dioxide, which is the waste product of metabolism. Through the vena cava, the oxygen-depleted blood goes into the right atrium and pumps into the right ventricle.

- Through the pulmonary artery, the right ventricle pumps the oxygen-depleted blood to the lungs, wherein carbon dioxide is removed and oxygen is replaced.

- The cycle starts again.

Just like any muscle in the body, the heart needs nutrients and oxygen in order to function. The arteries supply nutrients and oxygen that come from the aorta. These vessels open up to provide all areas of the heart with blood that is rich in oxygen.

The heart can be electrically divided into top and bottom chambers. An electrical impulse is produced in the top chambers of the heart, and causes the atria to squeeze and pump blood into the bottom chambers, where the ventricles are. A short pause happens to let the ventricles to fill. Then, the ventricles contract (beat) in order to pump blood to the lungs and the body.

Conducting System of the Heart

Sinoatrial node or SA node, located in the right atrium, is the natural pacemaker of the heart. The SA node functions independently from the brain, or without external control to produce electrical impulses for the heart to beat.

- The electricity produced by the SA node travels through the electrical grid of the heart, and sends signals to the atria's muscle cells to contract at the same time, making it possible for a synchronized squeeze of the heart. The atria pumps blood into the ventricles through contraction.

- The electrical signals produced in the SA node run through a junction box called the atrioventricular (AV) node, which is located between the atria and ventricles, where they are delayed for a couple of milliseconds to enable the ventricles to fill.

- Then, the electrical signals run through the ventricles and stimulate the heart muscle cells to contract. This ventricular contraction pushes blood to the lungs and the body.

- There is a short delay while the blood goes back to the heart before the electrical cycle starts again for the next heartbeat.

Chapter 2: EKG Basics

Electrocardiography is an important part of the assessment on the cardiovascular system. EKG is a valuable tool in examining heart arrhythmias and ischemia, as it shows the electrical activity of the heart.

Depolarization of the Heart

The depolarization of the heart muscle follows a certain route. The recurring electrical stimulus is produced at the SA node in the right atrium. With a rate of 60 to 100 beats a minute, the electrical stimulus causes waves of depolarization to run through the conducting pathways, causing the heart muscle to contract.

Stimulation begins at the atria, which contract almost at the same time. After that, the depolarization passes through the AV node where it pauses for a really brief period, before travelling into the Bundle of His. Then, it stimulates the Bundle Branches, and then runs through the ventricular muscles, causing contraction.

Depolarization that occurs in this sequence is considered as "In Sinus Rhythm," a rhythm that begins from the SA node.

Sodium ions run into the cell during depolarization. Afterwards, the calcium ions run into the cell, which cause muscular contraction. Lastly, the potassium ions flow out of the cell. Repolarization occurs as the ion concentration goes back to its pre-contraction condition.

Basic EKG Trace

- **P Wave**
  The P wave is related to contraction of the atria. It corresponds to atrial depolarization. Compared to the

ventricles, the atria have a small muscle mass, so P waves are also relatively small. A P wave must come first before every QRS complex.

- **QRS Complex**
  The QRS complex is related to the contraction of the ventricles. Compared to the P waves, the QRS complex is in large amplitudes.

- **PR Interval**
  The PR Interval is the part of the EKG trace between the start of the P wave and the start of the QRS complex. The length of the PR Interval is connected to the contraction of the atria, along with the distribution of depolarization through the conduction pathways to the ventricles.

- **ST Segment**
  The ST segment is the non-deflected part of the EKG trace between the S wave and the start of the T wave.

- **T Wave**
  The T wave is connected to the recovery or repolarization of the ventricles.

Timing, Speed, and Rate

Since all 12-lead EKG tests are standardized, their traces are calibrated in the same way. The speed of EKG/ECG paper is normally 25 mm/second, which means one large box represents 0.2 seconds, or 200ms.

To calculate the ventricular rate, use the interval between the adjacent R waves. To calculate the atrial rate, use the interval between the adjacent P waves. However, be careful because the P waves can sometimes be difficult to see.

<u>Intervals and Segments of the ECG</u>

The concepts of interval and segment may seem to be the same, but they are not. A segment is a line (normally isoelectric) that joins two waves. An interval is the part of the EKG that includes one or more waves, and a segment.

- **PR Interval** – this represents the physiological delay endured by the stimulus through the AV node. It is calculated from the start of the P wave to the start of either the Q or R wave (QRS complex). The normal value of the PR interval ranges from 0.12 seconds to 0.20 seconds. The PR interval can be shortened in cases like Pre-excitation Syndromes, so this denotes accelerated AV conduction. It can be prolonged in cases like First degree AV Block, which indicates AV conduction is delayed.

- **RR Interval** – this is the distance between two successive R waves. The RR interval must be constant in Sinus Rhythm. Its duration depends on the heart rate. It is calculated from the start of an R wave to the start of the next one.

- **QRS Interval** – this measures the whole duration of ventricular depolarization. It is calculated from the onset of either the Q or R wave to the end of the S wave. The normal value of the QRS interval ranges from 0.06 seconds to 0.10 seconds. This interval includes the set of waves comprising the QRS complex. It can be shortened by Pre-Excitation Syndromes, and prolonged by First Degree Heart Block.

- **QT Interval** – this represents the whole duration of ventricular depolarization and repolarization, or the electrical systole. It is calculated from the start of the Q wave to the end of the T wave. The normal value of the QT interval ranges from 340 ms to 450 ms in young adults, 470 ms in women, and 460 ms in children below 15 years old.

- **ST Segment** – this represents the interval or duration between ventricular depolarization and repolarization. It is calculated from the end of the S wave (QRS complex), and the start of the T wave. ST segment abnormalities are important for the proper diagnosis of Acute Coronary Syndromes.

ECG Electrodes

The electrical activity that goes through the heart is measured by external electrodes. These electrodes are attached to different areas of the body, and the activities from the electrodes are registered into the ECG.

All in all, there are 12 leads that are measured using the following 10 electrodes:

- Six chest electrodes
    - V1 – right of the sternum (4th intercostal space)
    - V2 – left of the sternum (4th intercostal space)
    - V3 – between V2 and V4
    - V4 – the nipple line or under the breast in women (5th intercostal space)
    - V5 – between V4 and V6
    - V6 – mid-axillary line, horizontal line from V4 (same level as V4)

- Four extremity electrodes:
    - RA – right arm
    - LA – left arm
    - F – left leg
    - N – neutral, right leg

    It does not matter whether the electrodes are attached distal or proximal on the extremities, but it is helpful to make this uniform. For example, do not put an electrode on the left wrist and one on the right shoulder.

12 leads can be obtained using these 10 electrodes. There are six precordial leads and six extremity leads.

Extremity Leads

The extremity leads record electrical activity transmitted into the frontal plane. The following are the extremity leads:

- Bipolar extremity leads
    - Lead I – left arm (+) to right arm (-)
    - Lead II – left leg (+) to right arm (-)
    - Lead III – left leg (+) to left arm (-)

- Unipolar extremity leads
    - aVR – right arm lead
    - aVL – left arm lead
    - aVF – left leg lead

    The "a" stands for augmented and the "V" stands for voltage.

Chest Leads

The chest or precordial leads record the electrical activity transmitted into the horizontal plane. These six leads are used to obtain information about the posterior and anterior parts of the heart. All of the chest leads are a unipolar lead.

ECG Variants

Aside from the standard 12-lead ECG, there are other ECG variants available:

1. **3-channel ECG** – this uses 3 or 4 electrodes. Yellow is used on the left arm, red on the right arm, black on the right leg, and green on the left leg. These basic leads obtain enough information to monitor the heart rhythm. However, these leads are inadequate to determine the ST elevation as none of the leads provides ST information regarding the anterior wall. If there are ST changes recorded using 3-channel ECG monitoring, this should prompt the use of a 12-lead EKG.

2. **5-channel ECG** – this uses 1 precordial lead and 4 extremity leads. This improves the accuracy of the ST segment, but the 12-lead ECG is still superior compared to this tool.

3. **Vector electrocardiography** – this tool is seldom used these days, but it still can be helpful in a research setting. It provides the spatial QRS-T angle generated from a computerized matrix operation. The three leads are X (right-left axis), Y (head-to-feet axis), and Z (front-back axis).

4. **Electrocardiographic body surface mapping** – this uses numerous leads (about 80 or more) to detect the electrical activity of the heart. Compared to the 12-lead ECG, using multiple leads may lead to improved diagnostic accuracy of acute coronary syndrome (ACS), or acute myocardial infarction (AMI).

Chapter 3: Types of Electrocardiograms

Resting 12-Lead EKG

The resting 12-lead EKG is the standard EKG/ECG test used in clinical settings today to measure the electrical functions of the heart. The patient lies still with 10 electrodes simultaneously attached to their chest, arms, and legs. The electrodes provide views from 12 different angles of the heart. This will help the doctor locate any abnormality in the heart function of the patient. A Resting 12-lead EKG is crucial for doctors to properly monitor a patient, and provide the right diagnosis.

Note that this test uses only 10 electrodes attached on the surface of the skin at different locations. One electrode is attached on each arm and leg, and the other six are attached on the chest. The 12 leads, or 12 views are obtained from the combination of electronic signals sent by the 10 electrodes to the EKG/ECG machine.

A routine checkup can include the Resting 12-lead EKG test to detect heart conditions before signs and symptoms start to show.

Holter Monitor

A Holter monitor is a small, wearable device used to continually monitor the EKG/ECG tracing for 24 to 48 hours. The electrodes are attached to the chest and wired into a recording device that can be carried in the pocket, or worn on a shoulder strap or a belt. The patient can perform their regular activities while wearing the Holter monitor as long as the electrodes and device stay dry. Additionally, the patient may be asked to keep a journal of the time and what they are doing when symptoms occur. The doctor will compare the electrical recordings to the diary to determine the reason for the symptoms.

Cardiac Event Recorder

The symptoms of a patient sometimes do not show during the Resting 12-lead EKG test or when using a Holter Monitor. If this is the case, the doctor may recommend a Cardiac Event Recorder that the patient can wear continuously for about 2-4 weeks. It is a portable, battery-operated device that the patient can control to record the electrical activities of the heart whenever they feel symptoms. Unlike the Holter Monitor, a Cardiac Event Recorder does not record the rhythm of the heart continuously.

- **Event Monitor** – a doctor may recommend to a patient to wear an event monitor if their symptoms do not occur often. It is similar to a Holter monitor as both of them are portable, but an event monitor only records at specific times and for just a few minutes every time. The device can either be worn on the wrist or be hand-held. The back of an event monitor has small metal discs that serve as the electrodes. It can be worn for a longer period than a Holter monitor, which is usually for 30 days.

  When a patient uses an event monitor, they can activate it by pressing a button to record when they feel any symptom or when their heart is beating at a fast rate. There are also other event monitors that automatically detect irregular heart rhythms and then begin recording.

  When a patient holds or wears an event monitor on their wrist, they will not need to attach electrodes on their chest. Instead, for a hand-held device, they would simply put it against their chest and press the record button, and for a device worn on the wrist, just press the record button when they experience any symptoms.

- **Loop Memory Monitor** – a compact device that can be attached to the skin surface surrounding the area of the heart. It records the EKG/ECG of a patient for a specific period of time (e.g. 5 minutes). To activate it, the patient simply need to push a button, and then it will store the EKG/ECG before and during the symptoms. For example, if the patient faints and pushes the button after recovering, the device will record the EKG/ECG during the time they felt dizzy and fainted, and right after they pushed the button. When the memory of the device is full, it will begin to overwrite the oldest recording.

An event recorder can fail to record the beginning of an irregular heart activity because of the delay in starting the record function. After pressing the record button, a loop memory monitor records the immediate few minutes before the onset of the irregular heart activity, keeps recording for a few more minutes, and then stops recording.

The device can be programmed to automatically record the event, or the patient can manually instruct it to start recording when they experience any symptoms.

The patient can wear a loop memory monitor for up to 30 days while still doing their regular everyday activities. They can remove the device when they shower or swim.

When using any of these two cardiac event recorders, the patient can send their EKG/ECG reading to a receiving or transmission center in the clinic, hospital, or doctor's office via telephone. The doctor will use these recorded electrical impulses to check the patient's heart rhythm during the time their symptoms occurred. If the EKG/ECG tracing suggests an emergency, the doctor will recommend the patient to immediately go to the emergency room.

Implantable Loop Recorder

Implantable loop recorder or ILR, also called insertable cardiac monitor, is a device similar to a Holter monitor in the sense that it continuously monitors the heart rhythms of the patient, but for a significantly longer period of time. IRL is just about the size of a USB memory stick or a pack of chewing gum.

Patients with unexplained episodes of syncope (fainting), dizziness, seizures, lightheadedness, or recurrent palpitations, and those who are diagnosed or at risk for atrial fibrillation are recommended to use an ILR. Like the loop memory monitor, the ILR can be set to automatically begin recording once an abnormality in the heart rhythm is detected. The patient can also carry around some kind of a remote control or a wrist band that serves as an external trigger to activate the device.

A minor surgery is performed to implant the ILR under the skin of the patient's chest, above the heart. This device is recommended for those who are experiencing symptoms that cannot be easily monitored within 30 days, which is the longest period of time that a cardiac event monitor can record. Because of its battery life of about 2-3 years, the device can be used to monitor the heart for an extended period.

Signal-averaged Electrocardiogram

A Signal-averaged electrocardiogram or SAECG is a special EKG/ECG test wherein multiple electrical EKG/ECG tracings are acquired over about 20 minutes to evaluate several hundred cycles of the heart, determining subtle abnormalities that increase the risk of heart arrhythmias. Arrhythmia is a medical condition that can cause cardiac arrest. The procedure is done similarly to a standard EKG/ECG, but it utilizes advanced technology to evaluate the risk.

The standard EKG/ECG machine does not usually detect these subtle abnormalities. The Signal-average ECG uses a computer to obtain all of the electrical activity of the heart, and to average them in order to show the doctor further information about how the electrical conduction system of the heart is functioning.

The test is done while the patient is lying down as motionless as possible, breathing normally, and not talking because the computer is quite sensitive to coughing, turning, and movements. The doctor or medical technologist will put the electrodes on the patient's chest and back to obtain electrical signals from the heart. A special EKG/ECG device will amplify and average the electrical signals until practically all noise is removed. The computer will evaluate about 500 heartbeats of the patient, and then the doctor will interpret the results.

SAECG recording produces an averaged QRS potential, normally printed on a scale much larger than a standard ECG, wherein SAECG makes calculations to show small variations in the final part of the QRS complex. This information can be interpreted right away by comparing findings with cut-off values.

Stress Test

A Stress Test is also called an exercise EKG, treadmill test, or cardiac stress test. If a patient most often feels their symptoms during exercise, the doctor will ask them to pedal a stationary bike or walk on a treadmill during an EKG/ECG. The treadmill is usually recommended for patients that can walk. There will be connections between the patient and an EKG monitoring machine. As the test continues to progress, the physical activity will increase in intensity.

If a patient has a walking disability, a hand pedaling stationary bike will be recommended for them. If a medical condition makes it difficult for them to exercise, the doctor may give them a medication that creates the same effect that exercise does to their heart.

The Stress Test is designed to evaluate how the heart of the patient can handle additional external stress. If the EKG detects any abnormalities during the test, those can be a sign of underlying heart disease.

This test is beneficial for the overall evaluation of an individual's health. It is often used by certain professionals, such as astronauts and aviators, for their routine health checkups.

Chapter 4: When Do You Need Electrocardiogram?

Reasons for Having an EKG/ECG

An EKG/ECG is a common heart test and is the only way to determine certain problems with the electrical impulses of the heart. Aside from providing information about the rate and rhythm of the heart, an EKG/ECG can also show if hypertension or high blood pressure caused an enlargement of the heart or if there is a presence of myocardial infarction or heart attack. Even if a heart attack is not present, the EKG/ECG test can help determine whether the pain is because of atherosclerosis (a buildup of plaque in the arteries), or angina (chest pain or discomfort when the heart muscle does not receive enough oxygen-rich blood).

An initial EKG/ECG test may show normal results even if the patient has a heart disease. A series of tests may be required over time to see an abnormality.

An EKG/ECG test provides two major types of information. First, a doctor can find out how long it will take for the electrical wave to pass through the heart once they measure the time intervals on the EKG/ECG. This information will show whether the electrical activity is slow, fast, irregular, or normal. Second, a cardiologist can determine if there are areas of the heart that are overworked or too large once they measure the amount of electrical activity that passes through the heart muscle.

When Do You Need EKG/ECG?

It is necessary in some cases to get an EKG/ECG test. The people who may need an EKG/ECG test are those who are experiencing signs and symptoms like the following:

- Chest pain
- Shortness of breath when tired

- Rapid pulse
- Irregular heartbeat
- Heart palpitations
- Fatigue
- Weakness or a decrease in ability to exercise
- Lightheadedness, dizziness, or confusion

Those who have risk factors for having a heart disease like high blood pressure are also recommended to take an EKG/ECG. In addition, a patient may also need this test if their family has a history of diabetes, heart disease, and other risk factors, or if they already have a heart disease. Some people take the EKG/ECG test for screening or work-related requirements.

Doctors may use an EKG/ECG to detect the following:

- A previous heart attack
- Abnormalities in the heart rhythm (arrhythmias)
- Structural problems with the chambers of the heart
- If coronary artery disease (narrowed or blocked arteries in the heart) is causing a heart attack or chest pain
- How well some heart disease treatments are working

When Do You Not Need EKG/ECG?

An EKG/ECG test may not be helpful in routine checkups for those who do not have symptoms of a heart disease, such as chest pain, or risk factors for a heart disease like high blood pressure. However, many people with no symptoms or risk factors take an EKG/ECG test for their routine checkups. A heart disease can be prevented through other more effective means than routine EKG/ECG tests. While the EKG/ECG is not harmful, it can sometimes indicate mild nonspecific irregularities that are not caused by an underlying heart disease. This can lead a person to worry and have follow-up tests, treatments, and medications that they do not need.

How to Protect the Heart

Whether a person has a heart disease or simply wants to prevent it, the following steps can help protect the heart.

1. **Know the risks** – a health care provider will be able to assess if a person has risk factors. The risk of having a heart disease depends on several factors, such as blood pressure, sex, age, cholesterol, ethnicity, or if the person smokes or has diabetes.

2. **Reduce the risks** – the following are the best ways to reduce the risk of a heart disease:

   - Do not smoke
   - Be aware of the risks
   - Control your blood pressure
   - Control your blood cholesterol
   - Exercise or be physically active
   - Attain a healthy weight and maintain it
   - Reduce stress
   - Limit alcohol use
   - Manage your diabetes
   - Regularly visit a health care provider and follow their advice
   - Eat a healthy diet

3. **Test your blood pressure** – use a blood pressure cuff to measure your blood pressure at least once a year. A doctor will recommend the blood pressure to be tested more often for people who have high blood pressure or any related condition. You can ask your doctor regarding how often to have your blood pressure tested.

4. **Test your blood sugar** – people who are 40 years old and above need to have their blood tested every three years to check their blood sugar (glucose). Excessive amount of glucose can harm the blood vessels. Moreover, pregnant women and those with risk factors for diabetes must also have a blood sugar test. Ask your doctor

whether or not you need to have your blood sugar levels tested.

5. **Test your cholesterol** – a blood test for cholesterol is recommended for the following:

    - Men over 40 years old
    - Women over 50 years old or post-menopausal
    - Men with a waistline of over 40 in (102 cm)
    - Women with a waistline of 35 in (88 cm)
    - People with a heart disease, high blood pressure, or diabetes
    - People who have suffered from a stroke
    - Anyone who has a family history of stroke or a heart disease

    A doctor can recommend how often a person must have their cholesterol tested.

If your blood pressure, blood sugar, or blood cholesterol is too high, a doctor can help you lower them. A lot of people can manage diabetes and lower blood pressure and cholesterol by taking medicines and changing some aspects of their lifestyle. This lowers the risk of strokes and heart attacks.

Chapter 5: Calculating the Heart Rate

Heart rate can be easily calculated by taking a pulse, but an electrocardiogram might be needed to find out the size and location of the heart chambers, if the heart is beating normally, if the heart has any damage, or how well a drug or device is working. An EKG/ECG may also be done to check for heart problems or disease and to determine if a person's heart is healthy enough for an operation.

Method 1: Calculate the Space between QRS Complexes

1. Know what a normal "wave form" looks like on an ECG trace to let you see what part of the ECG corresponds to one heartbeat. You can calculate the heart rate through the length of a heartbeat. A normal heart beat has a P wave, QRS complex, and ST segment. To calculate the heart rate, the easiest one to use is the QRS complex.

   - The P wave corresponds to atrial depolarization or the electrical activity of the upper chambers of the heart (atria). It is a small semi-round shape located before the QRS complex.

   - The most visible part of the ECG trace is the tall QRS complex. It is quite easy to recognize as it is normally pointed, resembling a tall, thin triangle. It corresponds to ventricular depolarization, or the electrical activity of the lower chambers of the heart (ventricles).

   - The ST segment comes after the QRS complex. It is the flat portion before the other semi-round shape on the ECG (T wave). The ST segment provides vital information about certain things like potential heart attacks.

2. Find the QRS complex. As mentioned above, the QRS complex is usually the most recognizable of the patterns on the ECG. When a person has normal heart function, the QRS complex looks like a skinny and tall spike that happens repeatedly with the same rate throughout the ECG trace. When one QRS complex happens, it indicates that one heartbeat has occurred. Hence, the distance between QRS complexes can be used to calculate the heart rate.

3. Calculate the distance between QRS complexes (R-R interval). Determine how many large squares separate one QRS complex to the next QRS complex. Normally, an ECG has both large and small squares, so make sure the large squares are the reference point. Note how many large squares are in between the peak of a QRS complex and the peak of the next QRS complex.

   - It will often be a fractionated number because the QRS complexes will not settle precisely on the squares. For example, 3.4 squares may separate two QRS complexes.

   - A large square normally has 5 little squares, so the space between QRS complexes can be estimated to the nearest 0.2 units.

4. Use this formula to calculate the heart rate: 300/(number of large squares). For example, the number of large squares between QRS complexes is 3.4. 300/3.4 = 88.24. Round it off to the nearest whole number. The heart rate is 88 beats a minute.

   - The rate of a normal heart function is between 60 and 100 beats a minute. This can help you find out if you are on the right track with your calculations.

   - Note that 60-100 beats a minute is just a loose parameter. Some athletes who are physically fit and have a healthy heart may have a lower resting heart rate.

- Some diseases may also cause unhealthy slower heart rates (bradycardias), and some can result in an abnormally accelerated heart rate (tachycardias).

Method 2: Use the Six-Second Method

The six-second method is another fast and easy way to calculate the heart rate. This is also great for calculating heart rates for abnormal rhythms. When you are using this method, remember that you should count exactly 30 large squares, which is equal to 6 seconds.

1. Draw a line near the left side of the ECG paper. From that line, count 30 large squares and draw another line after that.

2. Count how many QRS complexes are there between the two lines.

3. Take that number and multiply it by 10. Remember that 30 large squares are equal to 6 seconds, so multiplying it by 10 will represent the number of heartbeats in 60 seconds or 1 minute. For example, if you have 9 QRS complexes within the 30 large squares, then 9 x 10 = 90 beats a minute.

Using the first method given above, calculating the space between QRS complexes can be effective for a regular heart rate. The space between these QRS complexes is most likely the same for a person with regular heart rate.

On the other hand, the six-second method is effective for determining the heart rate for people with abnormal heart rhythms. The QRS complexes in an abnormal heart rate are at irregular distances from each other. The six-second method provides an average on the distance between heartbeats, which is a more accurate number.

Chapter 6: How to Read an EKG

The EKG tracing is normally printed on paper for easier evaluation. It provides an outline of the electrical activity of the heart.

Heart Rate

As described in the previous chapter, an easy way to calculate the rate of a normal heart is to count the number of large squares between two QRS complexes, then divide 300 by that number. For example, there are 5 large squares between two QRS complexes: 300/5 = 60 heartbeats a minute.

However, if the heart rhythm is irregular, this method of calculating the heart rate does not work, and so a different method is needed.

- Count 30 large squares and count the number of QRS complexes inside those squares (equivalent to 6 seconds).

- Multiply that number by 10 to provide the average number of QRS complexes in one minute.

For example, if there are 6 QRS complexes within 30 large squares: 6 x 10 = 60 heartbeats a minute.

A normal adult heart rate is 60 to 100 beats a minute. Tachycardia is a heart rate that is more than 100 beats a minute and bradycardia beats below 60 a minute.

Heart Rhythm

A heart rhythm or sinus rhythm is described as having properly oriented O waves on the ECG. Normal sinus rhythm or NSR is sometimes used to refer to a particular type of sinus rhythm wherein the other areas on the ECG are within the normal limits. However, other types of sinus rhythms can be completely normal in certain clinical contexts and patient groups. Therefore, normal sinus rhythm can be a misleading term and using it is sometimes discouraged.

Map out several consecutive QRS complexes on the ECG paper, and then check if the succeeding QRS complexes are the same. Calculate the R-R intervals on the ECG to evaluate if the heart rhythm is regular or irregular.

Cardiac axis

Cardiac axis, also called the QRS axis, is the general direction of depolarization as it flows through the ventricles. The cardiac axis of a healthy person must be between -30 and +90 degrees.

Looking at leads I, II, and III will help you determine the cardiac axis. A positive deflection can be seen in all of these leads, but lead II is the most positive in a normal cardiac axis. The most negative deflection can be seen in aVR.

The direction of depolarization in right axis deviation becomes distorted to the right. The right area of the heart generates a stronger signal from an extra heart muscle. This forces lead I to become a negative deflection and lead III/aVF becomes a more positive deflection.

Right axis deviation is linked with pulmonary conditions because of the strain placed on the right area of the heart. However, this can be a normal reading in extremely tall individuals.

The direction of depolarization in left axis deviation is distorted to the left. This makes lead III have a negative deflection. It will be considered significant if lead II also has a negative deflection. Conduction defects usually cause left axis deviation.

P Waves

Look at the P waves in the EKG. Check that every P wave is followed by a QRS complex. Determine if the P waves look normal by checking their duration, shape, and direction.

If the P wave is not present, check whether there is any atrial activity, such as a chaotic baseline, sawtooth baseline, or no atrial activity at all.

PR Interval

The PR interval extends from the start of the P wave until the start of the QRS complex. Its duration is normally between 120-200ms.

QRS Complex

You need to evaluate these aspects of the QRS complex:

- Width – a narrow QRS complex (<0.12 seconds) happens when the electrical impulse is conducted from the Purkinje fiber and the Bundle of His to the ventricles. This causes a synchronized, well-organized ventricular depolarization. An example of this is an atrial ectopic beat wherein there is an extra heartbeat from the atria caused by abnormal electrical focus.

  A broad QRS complex (>0.12 seconds) happens when there is a sequence of abnormal depolarization. An example of this is an ventricular ectopic beat in which there is an extra heartbeat that originates from the ventricles.

- Height – a small QRS complex is defined as <10mm in the chest leads and <5 mm in the limb leads.

A tall QRS complex suggests ventricular hypertrophy, but this can also be because of body habitus, such as tall, slim people.

- Morphology – you have to evaluate the different waves of the QRS complex.
    - o Q waves – a pathological Q wave is 25% greater than the size of its succeeding R wave or >40ms in width and >2mm in height. Isolated Q waves can be considered normal. A single Q wave is generally not a cause for concern, but check for the Q waves in a whole area for evidence of a previous myocardial infarction. Q waves in V1-V2 and a T wave inversion is indicative of a previous myocardial infarction.

    - o Delta wave – this is an indistinct upstroke in the QRS complex. It indicates that the ventricles are stimulated at an earlier time than normal the AV node. The early stimulation slowly runs across the myocardium.

    - o R and S waves – check for R wave progression in V1-V6. V3 or V4 is where the transition from S-R wave to R-S wave must happen. Poor progression can be indicative of a previous myocardial infarction, but it can also happen in extremely large people because of lead position.

    - o J Segment – this is at the end S wave and start of the ST segment. The J point can be elevated causing the succeeding ST segment to be elevated as well. This is known as "High take off," a normal variant that can result in confusion because it looks like ST Elevation.

ST Segment

The ST segment is where the end of the S wave joins the start of the T wave. This line must be isoelectric on the EKG on a healthy individual.

- ST elevation – greater than 1mm in 2 or more adjacent limb leads or greater than 2mm in at least 2 chest leads.

- ST depression – greater or equal to 0.5mm in 2 adjacent leads.

T Waves

The T waves represent recovery or repolarization of the ventricles.

- Tall T waves – greater than 10mm in the chest leads and greater than 5mm in the limb leads.

- Inverted T waves – inverted T waves are normal in V1 and an inverted T wave in lead III can be a normal variant.

Chapter 7: Electrocardiogram and Heart Function

Electrodes attached on the chest wall can detect electrical impulses that the heart generates. Multiple leads provide various electrical views of the heart. The physician will interpret the EKG/ECG tracing and will learn about the patient's heart rate and rhythm, as well as (indirectly) the blood flow to the ventricles.

The term used for how fast the heart beats is called "rate." The electrical impulse that the SA node normally produces is 60 to 100 beats per minute. A heart rate that is under 60 beats per minute is described as bradycardia (brady means slow, cardia means heart), while a heart rate that beats over 100 per minute is called tachycardia (tachy means fast).

The type of heartbeat is called "rhythm." The heart beats normally in a sinus rhythm with every electrical impulse that the SA node generates, leading to a heartbeat or ventricular contraction. There are normal electrical rhythms, some are abnormal, and some are possibly life-threatening. A number of electrical rhythms are not generating a heartbeat and could be the cause of sudden death.

Normal and Abnormal Heart Rhythms

A normal heart for adults beats around 100,000 times a day. A normal resting heart beats around 60 to 100 times a minute, but a heart rate of 40-90 times a minute is still considered to be normal. During sleep, the heart rate falls naturally (as low as 30 beats a minute in young individuals) and it increases with emotion and exercise.

Normal or Sinus Rhythm

Sinus rhythm refers to a normal heart rhythm. It is named as "sinus" rhythm because of the fact that a normal heart rhythm comes from the natural pacemaker of the heart – the sinus node.

The chambers of the heart are comprised of millions of cells that are really small and cannot be seen without a microscope. These heart cells must contract in a coordinated manner. The cells in the atria should contract all together, and then after a fraction of a second, the cells in the ventricles should also contract so that the heart can pump blood properly. If the heart cells contract individually instead of together, the chambers of the heart will wiggle and the contraction will not be effective.

Abnormal Heart Rhythms or Arrhythmias

Abnormal rhythms of the heart are called arrhythmias. Heart arrhythmia is also known as cardiac dysrhythmia or irregular heartbeat. It is a set of heart conditions where the heart may beat irregularly, too slowly, too fast, or too early.

An abnormal flow of electrical impulses in the heart can cause arrhythmias. Electrical short circuit often causes electrical abnormality. Some people experience these electrical short circuits from birth, but others may develop a heart disease later in life that can cause short circuits. Some conditions that can cause short circuits include coronary artery disease, cardiomyopathy (heart muscle diseases), high blood pressure, lung disease, diseases of the thyroid, problems with the heart valves, sleep apnea, and many others.

Arrhythmias are usually divided into these categories:

- Irregular heartbeat – fibrillation or flutter
- Early heartbeat – premature contraction
- Fast heartbeat – tachycardia
- Slow heartbeat – bradycardia

Most cases of arrhythmias are not really serious, but some conditions can predispose the patient to cardiac arrest or stroke. If the arrhythmia is exceptionally abnormal, or caused by a damaged or weak heart, it can cause severe or potentially fatal symptoms.

Causes of Arrhythmia

Arrhythmia can be caused by any interruption to the flow of electricity that makes that heart contract. As mentioned, a healthy resting heart has a heart rate of 60-100 beats per minute. The healthier an individual is, the lower their heart rate when resting as a general rule. For example, the resting heart rate of Olympic athletes will normally be below 60 times a minute as their hearts are quite efficient.

There are several factors that can cause the heart to not work properly, including:

- Heart disease, such as congestive heart failure
- Diabetes
- High blood pressure (hypertension)
- Hyperthyroidism
- Excessive coffee consumption
- Smoking
- Drug abuse
- Alcohol abuse
- Mental stress
- Structural changes of the heart
- Scarring of the heart
- Some medications
- Some herbal treatments
- Some dietary supplements

A healthy individual almost never suffers from long-term arrhythmia, except if there is an external trigger, such as an electric shock or drug abuse. However, an underlying problem may cause the electrical impulses not to travel through the heart properly, which can increase the possibility of arrhythmia.

Different Types of Arrhythmia

Conduction of the electrical impulse can sometimes be delayed in any part of the system, such as the AV node, SA node, ventricles, or the atria. There are aberrant electrical impulses that can cause normal heart rhythms, but some can possibly be dangerous.

Bradyarrhythmias

Bradyarrhythmias are conditions with slow heart rhythms, which can be caused by a disease in the electrical system of the heart. When this happens, the individual may feel like they are going to faint, or they may actually collapse. Certain medications can also cause bradyarrhythmias. These conditions include a number of heart rhythm problems, such as atrioventricular conduction blocks and sick sinus syndrome.

There are various clinical presentations that range from asymptomatic ECG findings to a broad range of symptoms like central nervous symptoms, syncope, heart failure symptoms, or chronic and nonspecific symptoms like fatigue or dizziness.

It is extremely important to have a proper diagnosis for bradyarrhythmias including a symptom-rhythm correlation. This is generally determined using noninvasive diagnosis studies, such as an ECG. Bradyarrhythmias rarely involve invasive electrophysiologic testing. If underlying treatable conditions are ruled out, or if the condition is caused by reversible extrinsic factors, such as certain medications (glycosides, calcium channel blockers, or beta-blockers), cardiac pacing may be recommended as a therapy method in treating symptomatic bradyarrhythmias.

Atrioventricular Blocks

Atrioventricular Blocks or AV Blocks are a set of conditions affecting the conducting system of the heart that cause interruption or delay on the electrical stimulus between the atria and the ventricles. Alteration in the Bundle of His, or in the AV node can cause AV blocks, but metabolic alterations or malfunctions in other heart structures can also cause these conditions.

Types of AV Blocks

1. First Degree Atrioventricular Block

This condition is also called PR prolongation. In a First Degree AV block, the PR interval is prolonged beyond 0.20 seconds. The stimulus is delayed as it moves through the His-Purkinje system or the AV node, causing a delay for the QRS complex to appear.

The distinct alteration on the EKG/ECG is the lengthened PR interval and a narrow QRS complex if there is no other alteration present. Moreover, there is no interruption of AV conduction in First Degree AV Block, so as opposed to other types of AV blocks, every P wave is followed by a QRS complex.

2. Second Degree Atrioventricular Block

In this condition, the conduction of atrial impulse to the His Bundle and/or AV node is blocked or delayed. The EKG/ECG shows non-conducted P waves that are not followed by a QRX complex.

Classification of Second Degree Atrioventricular Block

A. Second Degree Atrioventricular Block, Type 1 – this is also called Wenckebach or Mobitz 1. There is a progressive slowing of the PR interval until the atrial impulse is totally blocked and stops generating a QRS electrical impulse.

When the P wave is blocked and there is no QRS produced, the cycle starts over with the progressive prolongation of the PR interval. Having a regular atrial rhythm is one of the main distinctive features of this condition.

Possible causes:

- Cardiac surgery
- Myocarditis caused by infections
- Myocardial infarction
- Medications that prevent AV node conduction, such as beta-blockers, digoxin, amiodarone, and calcium channel blockers
- Hypoxemia
- Increased vagal tone (athletes)
- Conditions that stimulate vagal tone

B. Second Degree Atrioventricular Block, Type 2 – also called Hay or Mobitz 2, this condition is less frequent compared to the abovementioned and usually suggests underlying Cardiac Pathology.

It can be distinguished by the following features:

- Non-conducted P waves
- No PR prolongation before P waves
- Fixed PR interval
- QRS complex is likely wide

This condition is clinically significant as it can quickly develop into complete heart block. Structural problem to the conducting system of the heart usually causes this rhythm. This structural problem may be caused by any of the following:

- Myocardial infarction
- Cardiac surgery
- Hyperkalemia
- Idiopathic fibrosis
- Autoimmune diseases that affect the heart

- Infections and inflammatory conditions

This condition must be treated with immediate transvenous pacing or transcutaneous pacing as there is a possibility that electrical impulses will not reach the ventricles and generate ventricular contraction.

If immediate TCP cannot be carried out or if it needs time to initiate TCP, Atropine could be attempted, but it must not be relied upon. Atropine must be avoided if myocardial ischemia occurs.

3. Third Degree Atrioventricular Block

Also called Complete Heart Block (CHB), Third Degree AV Block is a condition wherein the AV conduction is completely interrupted. It occurs when the electrical impulses that tell the heart when to beat do not pass between the atria and the ventricles as they should. To keep the ventricles beating, a backup system takes over, but the heart rate will be extremely slow compared to normal. This may affect the blood flow to the brain and body.

Sick Sinus Syndrome

Sick sinus syndrome, also known as sinus node dysfunction or sinus node disease, is a group of arrhythmias or heart rhythm problems wherein the sinus node is not correctly functioning.

The sinus node is a region of specialized cells in the right atrium that control the heart's rhythm. It usually generates a steady pace of normal electrical impulses. When a patient has sick sinus syndrome, these signals are irregularly paced.

In sick sinus syndrome, the heart rhythms of the patient can be interrupted by long pauses, too slow, too fast – or an interchanging combination of these heart rhythm problems. This condition is rare, but the risk of having it increases with age. A lot of patients with sick sinus syndrome later on need a pacemaker to maintain a regular rhythm of the heart.

These are the types of sick sinus syndrome:

1. Bradycardia-tachycardia syndrome – this condition causes the heart rate to alternate between abnormally slow and fast rhythms, often with a long pause between heartbeats.

2. Sinus arrest – the activity within the sinus node pauses and this causes skipped beats.

3. Sinoatrial block – the heart has an abnormally slow heart rate caused by electrical signals moving too slowly across the sinus node.

Different conditions and diseases that cause damage or scarring to the electrical system of the heart can be the cause of sick sinus syndrome. Another cause could be scar tissue inflicted by a previous heart surgery, specifically in children. This condition can also be rarely caused by genetic factors.

Certain medications, such as beta blockers or calcium channel blockers used for treating high blood pressure, and even other conditions that cause the heartbeat to be faster or slower than normal can also cause sick sinus syndrome. In most cases, deterioration of the heart muscle due to age can make the sinus node not function properly.

Most people affected by this condition experience a few or no symptoms at first. In some cases, symptoms start and end abruptly. Some of the symptoms are:

- Palpitations
- Fatigue
- Chest pains
- Fainting or weakness
- Slower than normal pulse
- Lightheadedness or dizziness
- Shortness of breath

- Confusion

Sick sinus syndrome can happen at any age, including infancy. It usually develops after many years, so it is common in people 65 years and above. In rare cases, this heart rhythm problem can be linked to other conditions like muscular dystrophy and certain diseases that affect the heart.

Bundle Branch Block

Bundle branch block occurs when there is a block or delay along the pathway where electrical impulses travel through in order to make the heart beat. This condition sometimes makes it more difficult for the heart to efficiently pump blood throughout the body.

The blockage or delay can happen along the pathway that transmits electrical impulses to the right or left side of the ventricles. Bundle branch block may not require treatment, but when it does, the patient has to manage their health condition, such as heart disease, which caused bundle branch block.

Electrical impulses within the muscle of the heart normally give signal for the heart to beat. These impulses travel through a pathway, including the left and right bundles. If any of these bundles is damaged because of an underlying medical condition, such as heart attack, this can block the electrical signals and cause the heart to beat irregularly.

The cause of this condition depends on which bundle branch is affected. There is also a possibility that bundle branch block can happen without a known cause.

The causes of left bundle branch block include:

- Myocardial infarction
- High blood pressure
- Myocarditis – a bacterial or viral infection of the heart muscle

- Cardiomyopathy – stiffened, weakened, or thickened heart muscle

The causes of right bundle branch block include:

- Myocardial infarction
- Pulmonary hypertension (PH or PHTN) – high blood pressure within the pulmonary arteries
- Myocarditis
- Congenital heart disease – an abnormality of the heart that is present at birth, such as a hole in the wall that separates the atria and atrial septal defect.
- Pulmonary embolism – a blot clot located in the lungs.

Most people who have bundle branch block do not experience symptoms. In fact, some people who have this condition are not aware that they have bundle branch block.

People who have bundle branch block may feel symptoms, such as:

- Feeling like they're going to faint
- Fainting

The following are the risk factors for this condition:

- Underlying health conditions – having a heart disease or high blood pressure increases the risk of developing bundle branch block.
- Increasing age – this condition is more common in older people than the younger ones.

Atrial Fibrillation

Atrial Fibrillation is an irregular heart rhythm that causes the top chambers of the heart or the atria to contract abnormally. The blood in the body is not moving well, so it is possible to have a heart failure when the heart is no longer able to keep up with the body's needs. It can also cause the blood to pool inside the heart and form clots. A person can have a stroke if there is a blood clot in the brain.

The possible causes of Atrial Fibrillation include the following:

- Cardiomyopathy
- Heart disease caused by high blood pressure
- Congenital heart disease
- Past heart surgery
- Heart valve disease

Medications, such as theophylline, adenosine, and digitalis, can increase the chance of having Atrial Fibrillation. It can also be linked to genetics, infections, or caffeine, heavy alcohol, or drug use.

Patients with this condition may feel the following symptoms:

- Palpitations
- Lightheadedness or dizziness
- Weakness or fatigue
- Shortness of breath
- Chest pain

People with the following medical conditions may have higher chance of having Atrial Fibrillation:

- Sleep apnea
- Overactive thyroid gland
- Long-term lung disease

Atrial Flutter

Atrial Flutter is usually a problem where one area of the atria is not properly conducting, so the irregular conduction has a consistent pattern. This can happen in the first week after a heart surgery, or to people with a heart disease. It is caused by an abnormal circuit within the right atrium.

Atrial Flutter and Atrial Fibrillation are closely related, and these two types of arrhythmias can sometimes alternate from one to the other.

The types of Atrial Flutter are:

- Persistent atrial flutter – this type can be a permanent condition.
- Paroxysmal atrial flutter – this condition comes and goes. An episode of this type of atrial flutter can last for hours or days.

There is no definitive study about the causes of Atrial Flutter, but it can result from:

- Heart diseases or heart problems:
    o Hypertension
    o Abnormal heart valves
    o Ischemia
    o Hypertrophy
    o Cardiomyopathy
    o Open heart surgery

- Substances that alters the way the heart transmits electrical impulses:
    o Alcohol
    o Stimulants, such as amphetamines, cocaine, cold medicines, diet pills, and caffeine

- A disease in another part of the body that affects the heart:
    o Pulmonary embolism
    o Chronic obstructive pulmonary disease or COPD
    o Hyperthyroidism

Some people do not experience any symptoms with Atrial Flutter, but those who do describe them as:

- Anxiety
- Palpitations
- Shortness of breath

Those with lung or heart disease who have Atrial Flutter may experience the following more significant symptoms:

- Syncope
- Lightheadedness
- Chest or heart pains

Paroxysmal Supraventricular Tachycardia

Paroxysmal supraventricular tachycardia or PSVT is a form of supraventricular tachycardia. The cause of this condition is not yet known.

People who have PSVT do not feel any symptoms. If they do, symptoms may include shortness of breath, lightheadedness, chest pain, palpitations, and sweating. Episodes of PSVT begin and end suddenly.

Risk factors include psychological stress, caffeine, nicotine, alcohol, and Wolff-Parkinson-White syndrome, a condition that is often inherited from parents. The typical underlying mechanism entails an accessory pathway that leads to re-entry. EKG findings show a fast heart rate (usually 150 to 240 beats a minutes) and narrow QRS complexes.

Valsalva maneuver, a type of vagal maneuver, is often used for the initial treatment. Adenosine may also be attempted if other treatment is not effective and the patient has a normal blood pressure. In the case that adenosine is not effective, a beta blocker or calcium channel blocker may be used. Treatment may also involve synchronized cardioversion. Patients can avoid future episodes through catheter ablation.

The types of paroxysmal supraventricular tachycardia are:

1. Accessory pathway tachycardia – a rapid heart rate caused by an extra pathway between the atria and the ventricles. The electrical impulses that control the rhythm of the heart travel around the heart really quickly, so it makes the heart beat abnormally fast.

2. Atrioventricular nodal reentrant tachycardia (AVNRT) – is a form of abnormally fast heart rhythm. This condition originates from an area above the Bundle of His. AVNRT is the most common PSVT. About 75% of cases of this condition occur in women.

    AVNRT happens when a reentrant circuit builds inside or just next to the AV node. The circuit typically has two anatomical pathways: a slow pathway and fast pathway, which are both located in the right atrium. The location of the slow pathway is slightly posterior and inferior to the AV node, often next to the anterior border of the coronary sinus. The location of the fast pathway is usually just posterior and superior to the AV node. Both of these pathways are created from tissue that acts really like the AV node.

    The slow and fast pathways must not be mistaken as the accessory pathways that cause atrioventricular reciprocating tachycardia (AVRT) and Wolff-Parkinson-White (WPW) syndrome. The location of the slow and fast pathways of AVNRT is inside the right atrium, near or within the AV node. The pathways show electrophysiologic characteristics resembling the AV nodal tissue. The location of the accessory pathways that cause AVRT and WPW syndrome is in the AV valvular rings. They have electrophysiologic characteristics resembling the muscular tissue of the ventricles.

    People who have AVNRT may suddenly feel rapid regular palpitations. There is often no known provoking factor, but some affected people say that they develop symptoms after consuming caffeine or alcohol and while in stressful situations. In some cases, when the patient starts to feel a fast heartbeat, there will be a brief decline in blood pressure, so they may feel other symptoms like lightheadedness and dizziness. If they have underlying coronary artery disease and their heart rate is really fast, they may also experience chest pain similar to angina. AVNRT is not often life-threatening.

If the patient is experiencing symptoms while getting medical attention, the EKG may present typical changes that confirm the condition. For recurrent palpitations, a doctor may advise the patient to use a Holter monitor.

Atrioventricular Reciprocating Tachycardia

Atrioventricular reciprocating tachycardia (AVRT) or atrioventricular reentrant tachycardia is a form of abnormally fast rhythm of the heart. AVRT is commonly connected to Wolff–Parkinson–White syndrome, wherein an accessory pathway enables electrical impulses from the ventricles to go into the atria and trigger earlier than normal contractions that causes repeated activation of the AV node.

This condition involves two distinctive pathways: an accessory pathway and the normal AV conduction system. When AVRT happens, the electrical impulse runs in the normal way from the AV node through the ventricles. The electrical signal then pathologically runs back into the atria through the accessory pathway, which causes atrial contraction, and goes back to the AV node in order to complete the reentrant circuit. Once started, this may go into a cycle that causes the heart to beat abnormally fast.

The onset of AVRT could be due to a premature impulse of ventricular, atrial, or junctional origin.

Some of the symptoms of AVRT include the following:

- Palpitations

- Shortness of breath
- dizziness
- Fainting

Ventricular Tachycardia

Ventricular Tachycardia is an arrhythmia that results from abnormal electrical signals in the ventricles, which makes the heart beat faster than normal, usually around 100 beats or more per minute and become out of sync with the atria.

When this happens, it may cause the heart not to pump enough blood to the lungs and body since the chambers are not in sync with each other, or are beating so fast that they do not have time to properly fill.

Ventricular Tachycardia is caused by an interruption in the normal electrical system that controls the rate of the pumping action of the ventricles. There are lots of factors that can contribute to this problem, including:

- Cardiomyopathy
- Congenital heart conditions
- Lack of oxygen to the heart caused by tissue damage from heart disease
- An inflammatory disease that affect the skin or other tissues
- Imbalance of electrolytes
- Medication side effects
- Recreational drug abuse

In some cases, the main cause of Ventricular Tachycardia cannot be identified.

Some people who experience brief bouts of Ventricular Tachycardia might not feel any symptoms, but others might feel:

- Shortness of breath
- Seizures

- Dizziness
- Palpitations
- Lightheadedness
- Chest pain

More serious or sustained bouts of Ventricular Tachycardia might cause cardiac arrest or fainting.

Ventricular Fibrillation

Ventricular Fibrillation consists of really fast, irregular electrical impulses. This causes the ventricles to quiver rather than pump blood. A heart attack may sometimes trigger it, and it causes blood pressure to drop, stopping the blood supply to the vital organs in the body.

When a person experiences this arrhythmia, they can collapse within seconds, so it requires immediate medical attention. Ventricular Fibrillation is the most common cause of sudden cardiac death. Some of the emergency treatments include CPR or cardiopulmonary resuscitation shocks to the heart using an automated external defibrillator (AED).

The most common cause of Ventricular Fibrillation is a problem caused by a scar in the heart's muscle tissue due to a previous heart attack, or a problem in the electrical impulses running through the heart sustained after having a first heart attack. In some cases, Ventricular Fibrillation starts as Ventricular Tachycardia.

The most common symptom of Ventricular Fibrillation is loss of consciousness. Others experience the following:

- Rapid heartbeat
- Shortness of breath
- Dizziness
- Chest pain
- Nausea

Factors that can increase the risk of having Ventricular Fibrillation include:

- A previous heart attack
- Congenital heart disease
- Injuries that have damaged the heart muscle like electrocution
- Cardiomyopathy
- Significant electrolyte abnormalities
- Use of illegal drugs like methamphetamine or cocaine

Long QT Syndrome

Long QT syndrome or LQTS is an arrhythmia that can cause rapid, chaotic heartbeats. These fast heartbeats may cause sudden seizure or a fainting spell. In some cases, the heart can erratically beat for so long that it can cause sudden death.

A person can have a genetic mutation that can put them at risk of being born with congenital Long QT Syndrome. Acquired LQTS can be caused by certain medical conditions, medications, and imbalances of salts and minerals in the body (electrolyte abnormalities).

LQTS is a treatable condition, so people who have it may be advised to take medications in order to prevent an erratic heartbeat. Treatment for some people may include an implantable device or surgery.

A person who has LQTS should avoid some medications that can cause the condition. After completing treatment, they have high chances to live and thrive, even while still having LQTS. It is also possible for them to go back to recreational and competitive sports.

The heart normally circulates blood throughout the entire body during every heartbeat. The electrical impulses that are running through the heart control the contraction and pumping of blood and cause the heart to beat. After every heartbeat, the electrical system of the heart refreshes itself to prepare for the next heartbeat.

The heart muscle of a person with Long QT Syndrome takes longer than normal to refresh after a beat. This interruption in the electrical system is described as a prolonged QT interval.

While LQTS causes abnormalities in the electrical recharging system of the heart, the structure of the heart is normal. Abnormalities in the electrical system may be inborn, or acquired because of a medication or underlying medical condition.

There are two types of inherited LQTS:

1. Romano-Ward syndrome – this happens in individuals who inherit just one genetic variant from one parent.
2. Jervell and Lange-Nielsen syndrome – this is a rare and more severe form that usually happens earlier. In this condition, the child inherits genetic variants from both of their parents. Apart from having LQTS, they are also born deaf.

Medications than can prolong the QT interval and disrupt heart rhythm include the following:

- Diuretics
- Some antipsychotic and antidepressant medications
- Certain anti-nausea medications
- Antiarrhythmic medications (for maintaining normal heart rhythms)
- Some antibiotics
- Certain antihistamines

These are the people who might have a higher risk of LQTS:

- Children, teens, and young adults who have a history of cardiac arrest or have experienced unexplained seizures, fainting, or near drowning.

- Family members of children, teens, and young adults who have a history of cardiac arrest or have experienced unexplained seizures, fainting, or near drowning.
- First-degree relatives of individuals who have LQTS.
- People with low calcium, potassium or magnesium blood levels.
- Those who take medications that are known to trigger prolonged QT intervals.

Through the EKG/ECG tracing, the doctor can also find out information as to whether the heart muscles are properly conducting electricity. They will analyze the electrical waves to check if blood flow to areas of the heart muscle has decreased. The doctor can also learn if there is an acute blockage due to a heart attack or myocardial infarction. This is one of the reasons why a patient should take an EKG/ECG test as soon as they feel chest pain.

Chapter 8: Different Heart Conditions and Corresponding EKG Readings

An abnormal EKG can mean different things. An abnormality in an EKG is sometimes a normal variant of the rhythm of the heart, and does not necessarily affect the health. In other instances, an abnormal EKG can indicate a medical emergency, such as arrhythmia or myocardial infarction (heart attack).

Coronary Artery Disease

Coronary artery disease (CAD), also called ischemic heart disease, is a group of diseases that includes myocardial infarction, sudden cardiac death, stable angina, and unstable angina. CAD is characterized by the buildup of plaque in the inner walls of the heart arteries that leads to narrowing of the arteries, and a decreased blood supply to the heart. It is the number one cause of angina and myocardial infarction.

Chest pain or discomfort is a common symptom of CAD. The pain may also radiate to the jaw, shoulder, neck, back, or arm. It may occasionally feel like heartburn.

Arrhythmias, major Q waves, and ST-T patterns were found to be associated with a three times higher risk of coronary artery disease. Frequent premature heartbeats, lesser Q-waves, and ST-T patterns were found to be associated with almost twice higher risk.

Heart Attack

Myocardial infarction or heart attack happens when the supply of blood to the heart is reduced or stopped. This condition may not be fatal, particularly when the patient is given medical attention and treatment to manage the blockage as soon as the heart attack happens. However, they may have a damaged heart after the heart attack.

Chest pain or discomfort is the most common symptom, which can also travel into the jaw, shoulder, neck, back, or arm. It often occurs in the left side or center of the chest and lasts for several minutes. Other common symptoms include sweating, weakness, and severe shortness of breath.

In the EKG, the ST segment usually appears as flat. When a person is suffering from a serious heart attack, the ST segment may have a humped, raised appearance.

Angina

Angina manifests as chest pain that causes decreased blood supply to the heart. Blood transmits oxygen all throughout the body. If the heart is deprived of oxygen, it can have serious consequences.

Angina can be caused by atherosclerosis, the blockage or narrowing of the artery that supplies blood to the heart.

The pain of angina is typically in the chest, although it may also travel to the jaw, left arm, or shoulder. Some people who have angina may notice that the pain is connected to physical exertion and can be relieved by rest.

An angina attack can also be related to sweating and shortness of breath. Women may experience angina somewhat in a different way. Compared to men, women seem to have more pain in their middle back area and shoulder, and more jaw, throat, and neck pain. If the symptoms of angina quickly become worse and happen at rest, this could be a sign of an impending heart attack.

In an EKG, the ST segment dips down rather than being flat.

Cardiac Aneurysm

An anterior myocardial infarction without timely and sufficient reperfusion therapy may result in massive loss of myocardial tissue. This can weaken the anterior ventricle wall, which can cause local swelling of the anterior wall. A profound case of this condition is called cardiac aneurysm.

Cardiac aneurysm often has typical EKG attributes: persistent ST elevation and anterior Q waves. Because of the severely decreased ejection fraction, individuals with cardiac aneurysm may have a bad prognosis. They often experience heart failure and are in danger of suffering from sudden death because of ventricular fibrillation.

Cardiomyopathy

A group of diseases of the heart muscle is called cardiomyopathy. Some types are genetic, while others acquire this disease due to infection or other causes that need further investigation. A common type of this condition is idiopathic dilated cardiomyopathy, in which the heart is enlarged. Other types include hypertrophic (thickened heart muscle), dilated (heart enlarged), and ischemic (loss of heart muscle).

Dilated cardiomyopathy (DCM) is characterized by global myocardial dysfunction (40% decreased ejection fraction), and ventricular dilatation. Patients often experience symptoms of biventricular failure, such as ankle edema, dyspnea, fatigue, and orthopnea.

DCM is linked to high mortality because of ventricular dysrhythmias (sudden cardiac death), or progressive cardiogenic shock.

The common EKG associations with dilated cardiomyopathy include:

- Biatrial enlargement
- Left atrial enlargement – may develop into atrial fibrillation
- Left axis deviation
- Left bundle branch block
- Biventricular enlargement or left ventricular hypertrophy

- QRS complexes in V1-V4 have poor R-wave progression ("pseudo-infarction" pattern)
- Ventricular dysrhythmias
- Ventricular bigeminy and frequent ventricular ectopic beats

Pericardial Disease

Pericardium is the sac that covers the heart and it could be affected by various conditions like stiffness (constrictive pericarditis), inflammation (pericarditis), and fluid accumulation (pericardial effusion).

Several EKG findings are connected with tamponade. Low-voltalge QRS complex, sinus tachycardia, and the usual EKG results in acute pericarditis, including PR segment depression and extensive upward concave ST segment elevation, can all be seen in cardiac tamponade. A QRS amplitude of >0.5 mV in the limb leads, called low-voltage QRS complex, has been found to be resolved in a week after treatment for tamponade by anti-inflammatory medications or pericardiocentesis. Electrical pericardiocentesis – the alteration of axis between beats, or the QRS complex amplitude – is specific, but not quite sensitive for cardiac tamponade. Electrical alterans represent that the heart is in a swinging motion in pericardial fluid.

Valvular heart disease

The valves of the heart keep the blood flowing through the heart in the right direction. However, a range of conditions can result in valvular damage. Valves may not close properly (prolapse), leak (insufficiency or regurgitation), or narrow (stenosis). Some people may be born with valvular heart disease, or the valves may become damaged by some conditions, such as connective tissue disorder, rheumatic fever, infections, and certain radiation treatments and medications for cancer.

Early in the disease, the ECG findings may be normal or show LV hypertrophy. There may also be a presence of left axis deviation. Because of an early overload of LV volume, prominent Q waves can be observed in lead I, aVL and V3-V6. As the valvular heart disease advances, there is a drop in the prominent initial forces, but the sum of QRS amplitude increases.

Wolff–Parkinson–White Syndrome

Wolff–Parkinson–White syndrome or WPW syndrome is a congenital condition that involves an extra electrical pathway between the atria and the ventricles that causes a rapid heartbeat.

Episodes of rapid heartbeats are usually not life-threatening, but the person affected may have severe heart problems. Treatment can prevent or stop episodes of rapid heartbeats. Ablation, a catheter-based method, can often resolve the heart rhythm problems permanently.

Most people who have an extra electrical pathway do not experience rapid heartbeat. WPW syndrome is only discovered by accident during a heart test. WPW syndrome is often not dangerous, but doctors may recommend further tests before children with WPW syndrome can join in high-intensity sports.

The symptoms of WPW syndrome include:

- Palpitations
- Shortness of breath
- Anxiety
- Fainting
- Lightheadedness or dizziness
- Fatigue

An episode of really fast heartbeats can suddenly start and can last for several hours or just a few seconds. Episodes can occur while at rest or during exercise. Symptoms can be triggered by alcohol and caffeine or other stimulants in some people.

When a person with Wolff–Parkinson–White syndrome takes an EKG test, it can show delta waves or slurred upstrokes before the QRS complexes. The ECG can also exhibit as a narrow-complex supraventricular tachycardia or SVT.

Atrial Flutter

Flutter is recognizable on the EKG as this condition is a rhythmic tachycardia, or tachyarrhythmia that has heart rates in divisors of 300 bpm, with 150 bpm as the most common in patients. On the EKG, there are no existing P waves, but atrial waves that have "saw-tooth" pattern are seen with heart rates around 300 bpm.

Except with previous aberrant conduction or bundle branch blocks, the QRS complex in atrial flutter is narrow. It is arrhythmic in some cases, and the conduction could be variable. Because of that, it could be misidentified as atrial fibrillation, but it is distinguished by the "saw-tooth" waves.

The "saw-tooth" wave is an attribute of the atrial flutter, particularly identifiable in the typical atrial flutter. The morphology in the EKG leads is mainly negative.

The main feature of atrial flutter is a slow downward start, followed by a rapid downward stage changing into a fast rise, settling on top of the isoelectric line while joining at the start of the following wave.

It can usually be seen between the T wave and its succeeding QRS complex. Moreover, it normally causes waves of the isoelectrical segments, functioning as a diagnostic support in high heart rates,

The EKG characteristics of atrial flutter are as follows:

- Absence of P waves
- QRS similar to the previous one, except aberrancy.
- Regular rhythm with a heart rate around divisors of 300 (75 bpm, 100 bpm, 150 bpm)
- Waves in a saw-tooth pattern that have heart rates of approximately 300 bpm.

Atrial Fibrillation

The main characteristic of atrial fibrillation on the EKG is that is it arrhythmic. It has RR intervals that are irregular, and does not have any pattern. A chaotic atrial stimulus has no P waves, but small atrial waves, known as f waves, can be seen.

The Normal Conduction System is where the conduction to the ventricles occurs, so QRS complexes are narrow.

The EKG of atrial fibrillation will show the following:

- No P waves can be seen, but small irregular waves (f waves) may be present.
- Irregular RR intervals
- Narrow QRS complexes, resembling morphology to the QRS complex that can be observed during sinus rhythm.

Atrioventricular Nodal Reentrant Tachycardia

Atrioventricular nodal reentrant tachycardia or AVNRT is the most common paroxysmal supraventricular tachycardia in healthy hearts, making up 60% of cases. Women in their 40's usually exhibit this condition.

On the EKG, AVNRT will show the following characteristics:

- Common AVNRT: no P waves present
- Uncommon AVNRT: inferior leads have negative P wave after the corresponding QRS.
- Narrow QRS complexes with heart rate of 120 to 250 bpm.

Conclusion

Thanks again for choosing this book!

I hope you enjoyed learning about EKG/ECG interpretation!

If you enjoyed this book, please take the time to leave me a review on Amazon. I appreciate your honest feedback, and it really helps me to continue producing high quality books.